Paleo Diet Cookbook

For Diabetics

Delicious Recipes

For A Healthy Weight Loss

(Includes Alphabetic Index, Nutrition Facts

And Step-By-Step Instructions)

By

Barbara P. Trisler

www.MillenniumPublishingLimited.com

www.MillenniumPublishingLimited.com

Copyright ©2019

All rights reserved. Except as permitted under the U.S. Copyright Act of 1976, the scanning, uploading and distribution of this book via the Internet or via any other means without the express permission of the author is illegal and punishable by law. Please purchase only authorized electronic editions, and do not participate in or encourage electronic piracy of copyrighted material.

Disclaimer

This publication is designed to provide competent and reliable information regarding the subject matter covered. However, it is sold with the understanding that the author is not engaged in rendering medical or other professional advice. Laws and practices often vary from state to state and country to country and if medical or other expert assistance is required, the services of a professional should be sought. The author specifically disclaims any liability that is incurred from the use or application of the contents of this book.

Table of Contents

Introduction 7

Chapter 1 9
   Diabetes Type 1 and 2 9
      Type 1 Diabetes 9
      Type 2 Diabetes 9
      Gestational Diabetes 10

Chapter 2 12
   What is the Paleo Diet? 12

Chapter 3 13
   The Benefits of the Paleo Diet for Diabetics 13

Chapter 4 16
   Paleo Diet Foods to Eat and Avoid 16
      Foods to Eat on the Paleo Diet 16
      Foods to Avoid on the Paleo Diet 18

Chapter 5 20
   Tips for Getting Started on the Paleo Diet 20

Chapter 6 22
   Paleo Diet Recipes for Diabetics 22

Breakfast Recipes 24
      Blueberry Coconut Smoothie 25
      Tomato Basil Omelet 25
      Spiced Apple Walnut Muffins 26
      Ham and Red Pepper Frittata 27
      Pumpkin Protein Pancakes 28
      Strawberry Ginger Beet Smoothie 29
      Sweet Potato Breakfast Skillet 30
      Coco-Vanilla Chia Pudding 31
      Spinach and Mushroom Omelet 31
      Raspberry Kale Smoothie 32
      Light & Fluffy Banana Protein Pancake 33
      Creamy Avocado Walnut Smoothie 34
      Vegetable Egg White Omelet 34
      Cinnamon Coconut Flour Waffles 35
      Triple Berry Smoothie 36
      Mixed Vegetable Frittata 36
      Chocolate Almond Butter Smoothie 37

Lunch Recipes 39

    Curried Butternut Squash Soup 40

    Avocado Egg Salad 41

    Roasted Tomato Basil Soup 41

    Avocado Spinach Salad with Egg 42

    Apple Walnut Chicken Salad 43

    Hearty Beef and Vegetable Stew 44

    Cream of Broccoli Soup 44

    Chopped Chicken and Mango Salad 45

    Mushroom and Leek Soup 46

    Creamy Cucumber Dill Salad 47

    Lamb and Root Vegetable Stew 48

    Easy Chicken and Vegetable Soup 49

    Spiced Pumpkin Soup 50

Dinner Recipes 51

    Rosemary Roasted Chicken 52

    Thai Coconut Vegetable Curry 53

    Herb-Roasted Pork Tenderloin 54

    Balsamic Grilled Salmon 54

    Slow Cooker Pulled Pork 55

    Seared Scallops with Herb Butter 56

    Meatloaf with BBQ Sauce 57

    Herb-Crusted Lamb Chops 58

    Zucchini Pasta and Meatballs 59

    Chicken Tikka Masala 60

    Slow Cooker Balsamic Roast Beef 61

    Cajun Chicken and Veggies 62

    Easy Garlic Shrimp 63

    Bacon-Wrapped Turkey Breast 63

    Grilled Salmon with Mango Sauce 64

    Lemon Chicken with Broccoli 65

    Maple Country Style Pork Ribs 66

    Cilantro Lime Chicken 67

    Curry Grilled Pork Chops 68

Snacks & Desserts 69

    Baked Cinnamon Apple Chips 70

    Avocado Deviled Eggs 70

    Chocolate Chia Pudding 71

    Sesame Kale Chips 72

    Almond Butter Brownies 72

    Cinnamon Roasted Nuts 73

Lemon Blueberry Cupcakes 74
Grilled Balsamic Peaches 75
Maple Walnut Trail Mix 75
Coconut Almond Chia Pudding 76
Baked Beet Chips 77

Conclusion 78

Index 79

How To Get The Color Paperback Version 80

How To Get The Bonus Recipe Image Booklet 80

Introduction

All it takes is a quick glance at the magazine rack at your local grocery store to keep up with the latest fad diets. These days it seems like a new diet hits the shelves every week, always making lofty promises of weight loss and improved health. Unfortunately, many of these diets are not based on a foundation of scientific truth and any results they produce fade quickly. While many diets are not worthy of your consideration, there is one that is – the paleo diet. Whether you want to lose weight, improve your digestion, or boost your overall health, this is the diet to try.

Some people know of the paleo diet as the caveman diet because it is based on the type of diet our Paleolithic Era ancestors followed. Though you don't have to hunt or scavenge for food, you do need to adhere to certain rules if you're going to follow the paleo diet. This diet excludes processed carbs and refined sugars as well as dairy products, grains, and legumes. It might sound a little restrictive at first but, once you get used to it, you'll be free from the negative health effects caused by the average Western diet and you'll be feeling better than you ever have before.

The paleo diet is scientifically proven to provide a wide range of health benefits. If you're reading this book, there is one benefit you are probably most interested – reversing diabetes. Type 2 diabetes affects millions of people, many of which do not make even the slightest effort to control or reverse their condition. With a healthy diet and regular exercise, however, it is entirely possible to reverse this condition! The paleo diet is a diet that is typically high in lean protein and fiber but low in carbohydrates and fat – exactly the type of diet that will help you stabilize your blood sugar, improve your insulin sensitivity, and manage your diabetes.

For many, diabetes is a lifelong condition. With the help of the paleo diet, however, it is possible to reverse type 2 diabetes and manage type 1 diabetes, reducing your dependence on supplemental insulin. If you'd like to learn more about the paleo diet and its benefits for diabetes, simply turn the page and keep reading!

<u>Please Note</u> - There are two different version of this book – one with color pictures and another without pictures. This particular version has no pictures. This is because of the prohibitive cost of printing images in color. However, the version with pictures is available on Amazon. See the end of this book for more details.

If you can't afford it, don't worry. A bonus PDF image booklet is available for download. It shows each recipe in this book in full color. See the end of this book for details on how to get it.

Without further ado, lets get started!

Chapter 1

Diabetes Type 1 and 2

All of the food you eat contains nutrients like protein, carbohydrates, and fat. Each of these nutrients plays an important role in your total health and wellness and they also contain energy. Most of the food you eat can be broken down into glucose by your digestive system. From there, a hormone called insulin helps your body absorb and utilize that glucose as a source of energy. Insulin is produced in the pancreas and your production of insulin varies depending on the type of food you're eating and how easy it is to digest. Foods that digest quickly (simple carbohydrates like white rice or bread) have a greater impact on your blood glucose levels than foods that take longer to digest (complex carbohydrates like whole grains).

When you eat, the insulin produced by the pancreas helps to transport the glucose from food to your bloodstream then to your cells where it can be used as energy. If you eat too many foods that cause your blood sugar level to spike and to remain high, your body might become resistant to the effects of insulin – it will take more and more insulin to produce the desired effect. High blood sugar is the defining characteristic of diabetes, though there are several different types of diabetes. Here is a quick overview of each:

Type 1 Diabetes

This type of diabetes is an autoimmune condition in which the immune system accidentally attacks healthy cells in the pancreas, preventing it from producing insulin. This condition is usually diagnosed in childhood or early adolescence and it typically requires lifelong treatment with insulin.

Type 2 Diabetes

This type of diabetes is acquired and it can develop at any age. Type 2 diabetes typically develops when the body becomes resistant to the effects of insulin or if insulin production becomes impaired. This type of diabetes is particularly common in people who are overweight or obese and it can often be reversed if the patient improves his or her lifestyle.

Gestational Diabetes

This type of diabetes is seen in pregnant women and it often goes away after the baby is born. Having gestation diabetes increases your risk for developing type 2 diabetes later in life and sometimes type 2 is incorrectly diagnosed as gestational diabetes.

Diabetes affects nearly 30 million people in the United States – that's more than 9% of the American population. What's more, as many as 1 in 4 people who have diabetes don't even know it. In addition to obesity, other risk factors for diabetes include physical inactivity, family history of diabetes, race, high blood pressure, and other health problems. Treatment for diabetes generally involves taking supplemental insulin, though making healthy changes to your lifestyle can be beneficial as well.

When left untreated, diabetes can lead to some very serious complications including heart disease, kidney disease, nerve damage, eye problems, and stroke. Having diabetes can also reduce circulation to the extremities which, in some cases, leads to serious infections that eventually require amputation of the affected limb. Though there are differences between type 1 and type 2 diabetes, the symptoms of both are similar and may include:

- Excessive thirst
- Increased urination
- Extreme hunger
- Ketones in the urine
- Unexplained weight loss
- Fatigue
- Blurry vision
- Irritability
- Slow-healing of wound and sores
- Frequent infections

Diabetes can be a lifelong condition, though type 2 can potentially be reversed by making healthy lifestyle changes. For many people, losing weight by increasing physical activity and improving diet helps to reverse diabetes, though insulin treatments may still be needed while these changes are being put into effect. The best diet for someone with diabetes is a high-protein, high-fiber diet that is low in processed carbohydrates and moderate in healthy fats. Though you can certainly make these dietary changes on your own, many people find that the paleo diet works to improve their condition. You'll learn more about the paleo diet in the next chapter.

Chapter 2

What is the Paleo Diet?

There are countless fad diets out there that promise amazing results but many of them don't actually work or, if they do, the results are short-lived. The paleo diet is more than just a fad diet – it is a healthy lifestyle that involves eating wholesome, natural foods that have been largely unaltered by man. The name paleo diet comes from the Paleolithic Era when humans lived hunter-gatherer lifestyles. Agriculture had not yet been developed, so humans lived off the land, hunting game and gathering other edibles. The modern paleo diet is based on the idea that human genetics have not changed significantly since the Paleolithic Era and, therefore, humans are still biologically optimized for a diet made up of natural foods.

Following the paleo diet doesn't require you to hunt for your own food, but it does require you to think a little more carefully about your dietary choices. This diet is focused primarily on lean proteins, fresh fruits and vegetables, nuts, seeds, and healthy fats. The paleo diet excludes all processed foods and refined carbohydrates as well as dairy products, grains, and legumes. Essentially, the paleo diet includes foods that would have been available to our Paleolithic Era ancestors prior to the birth of agriculture. There is some wiggle room, of course, but that is the leading principle behind the diet. In the next chapter, you'll learn about the benefits of the diet.

Chapter 3

The Benefits of the Paleo Diet for Diabetics

The paleo diet is focused around wholesome, natural foods like lean meats and seafood, fresh fruits and vegetables, nuts, seeds, and healthy fats. As such, the paleo diet overlaps with aspects of certain other diets which have been linked to significant health benefits including the Mediterranean diet and the DASH diet.

Though many would call the paleo diet restrictive, it is actually much simpler to follow than you might think. You must cut out grains and dairy products, but that still leaves you with plenty of options. We'll go into greater detail about the foods that you can and can't eat on the paleo diet in a later chapter – for now, let's focus on the benefits of the paleo diet.

The benefits of the paleo diet are similar to the benefits of any diet that is developed around wholesome, natural foods. Here are some of the top benefits:

a) More lean muscle mass

The paleo diet is focused on lean proteins like grass-fed meat, free-run poultry, and wild-caught fish – all of these help you to build and maintain lean muscle mass.

b) Improved digestive health

Refined sugars and processed carbohydrates can cause inflammation in the intestinal tract which can impair your body's ability to properly digest and utilize nutrition from the foods you eat. Removing these foods will allow your digestive system to heal.

c) Increased longevity

Following a diet low in processed foods and saturated fat has been shown to increase lifespan – it also helps you to avoid chronic diseases which might shorten your lifespan.

d) Highly concentrated nutrition

The foods that are included in the paleo diet are naturally rich in nutrients – synthetic vitamins and minerals used to fortify processed foods are less biologically valuable than natural sources for the same nutrients.

e) Fewer allergies

The paleo diet is naturally free from some of the most common food allergens such as grains like corn and wheat – it is also free from dairy products.

f) Reduced inflammation

Chronic inflammation is a leading factor behind numerous diseases including cardiovascular disease. Many of the foods included in the paleo diet have anti-inflammatory benefits.

g) Increased energy levels

When you cut out foods that damage your digestive system and interfere with the absorption of nutrients, your body can begin to heal. As your digestion improves and you start absorbing nutrients once more, your energy levels will improve as well.

h) Healthy weight loss

Though the paleo diet isn't strictly low-calorie, many of the foods included are nutrient-dense and lower in calories than most processed foods. This diet can help you lose weight and keep it off.

i) Reduced risk for disease

Many of the most serious chronic diseases are, at least in part, related to an unhealthy diet. Improving your diet can help to reduce your risk for serious diseases.

In addition to the benefits already listed, the paleo diet is also particularly beneficial for people with diabetes. By removing refined sugar and processed carbohydrates from your diet, you can stabilize your blood glucose levels to avoid blood sugar spikes. Once your blood sugar stabilizes, your body can begin to repair and heal itself from insulin resistance, enabling you to once more digest and absorb nutrition from the food you eat.

The paleo diet can also help you to achieve and maintain a healthy bodyweight which will help you to prevent your diabetes from coming back once you successfully reverse it. Keep reading to learn about the specifics of the paleo diet.

Chapter 4

Paleo Diet Foods to Eat and Avoid

As you have already learned, the paleo diet is made up of wholesome, natural foods – foods that have been minimally altered by man. This includes lean proteins like grass-fed meats, free-run poultry, cage-free eggs, and wild-caught fish as well as fruits and vegetables. It also includes nuts, seeds, and healthy fats. Refined sugars and processed carbohydrates have no place in the paleo diet, nor do dairy products, grains, legumes, or white potatoes. To help you see exactly which foods are and are not allowed on the paleo diet, here are some helpful food lists:

Foods to Eat on the Paleo Diet

Proteins		
Bacon	Chicken	Eggs
Beef	Clams	Elk
Bison	Duck	Fish
Goose	Pork	Shrimp
Lamb	Quail	Turkey
Lobster	Rabbit	Veal
Pheasant	Scallops	Venison

Fruits & Vegetables		
Apples	Cherries	Onions
Apricots	Cucumber	Papaya
Asparagus	Eggplant	Parsnips
Artichoke	Grapes	Peaches

Arugula	Grapefruit	Pears
Bananas	Green beans	Pineapple
Beets	Guava	Plum
Bell peppers	Herbs	Pomegranate
Bok choy	Honeydew	Pumpkin
Blackberries	Kale	Raspberries
Blueberries	Kohlrabi	Spinach
Broccoli	Kiwi	Strawberries
Brussels Sprouts	Lemon	Sweet potato
	Lime	Swiss chard
Cabbage	Lettuce	Squash
Carrots	Leeks	Tomatoes
Cantaloupe	Mango	Turnips
Cauliflower	Mushrooms	Watermelon
Celery	Nectarines	Zucchini

Nuts & Seeds		
Almonds	Brazil nuts	Cashews
Chestnuts	Macadamia nuts	Sesame seeds
Chia seeds	Pecans	Walnuts
Flaxseeds	Pine nuts	Hazelnuts
Hemp seeds	Pumpkin seeds	Turkey

Healthy fats		
Avocados	Macadamia oil	Coconut oil
Olive oil	Ghee	Tallow
Grass-fed butter	Lard	Walnut oil

Other Foods		
Almond flour	Dark chocolate	Honey
Almond milk	Arrowroot powder	Maple syrup
Baking powder	Pepper	Salt
Baking soda	Cocoa powder	Spices
Coconut	Stevia	Coconut aminos
Tapioca starch	Coconut flour	Tea
Coconut milk	Vanilla extract	Coffee
Vinegar		

Foods to Avoid on the Paleo Diet

Fruits, Drinks & Vegetables		
Alcohol	Regular yogurt	Artificial sweetners
Ice cream	Baked goods	Lentils
Barley	Margarine	Beans
Oats	Bread	Pasta
Brown rice	Peanuts	Brown sugar

Peanut butter	Candy	White Potatoes
Canola oil	Quinoa	Cereal
Rye	Cheese	Soft drinks
Chickpeas	Soy beans	Corn
Soy sauce	Cornstarch	Split peas
Corn oil	Vegetable oil	Couscous
Wheat	Cow's milk	White rice
Cream cheese	White sugar	Energy drinks

N/B: This list is by no means complete but it gives you an idea what foods to look out for. Avoid all grains, dairy products, and legumes as well as processed foods and refined sugars.

Chapter 5

Tips for Getting Started on the Paleo Diet

The paleo diet is more a lifestyle than an actual diet – it incorporates certain dietary principles but also advocates for a healthy lifestyle in general. If you'd like to give the diet a try, there are some simple things you can do to ease yourself through the transition – here are some tips:

Start increasing your protein intake and reducing your carbohydrate intake – you should also be eating a moderate amount of healthy fats.

Swap fresh fruits and vegetables for grains and legumes – be sure to include some vegetables at every meal.

Replace hydrogenated oils with coconut oil or olive oil for cooking and limit your intake of saturated fats.

Stop using refined sugars like granulated sugar and brown sugar, swapping in natural sweeteners like honey and pure maple syrup.

Focus on healthy cooking methods like grilling, baking, broiling, and poaching instead of frying.

As you make these changes to your diet, you'll find that adhering to the principles of the paleo diet is not as difficult as you once imagined. When shopping for groceries, take the paleo food list from the previous chapter with you so you know what to look for.

Generally speaking, however, most of the foods you find in the outer aisles at the grocery store are safe – things like fresh produce, meat, and seafood. If you're going to commit to the paleo diet, you might want to start by cleaning out your pantry of all non-paleo foods and then stock up on approved foods so you have plenty of options.

Just because you're following the paleo diet doesn't mean that you can't enjoy food. Fresh herbs and dried spices are all included in the diet and can be used to add flavor to your favorite paleo dishes. You can also continue to eat out while following the paleo diet, though you might have to order different dishes than you're used to. Dishes that feature grilled meats, salads, and many other entrees are already made with paleo-friendly ingredients or they can be made paleo with some minor adjustments. If you don't see something on the menu that fits the paleo diet, you can always order a green salad with grilled chicken or fish.

As you transition into the paleo diet, you may experience some withdrawal symptoms that result from cutting grains out of your diet. Fortunately, these symptoms usually only last a few days for most people. During this time, be sure to drink plenty of water and make sure to get adequate rest as well. It is also a good idea to make small changes over time instead of going cold-turkey on everything. The more gradually you make changes to your diet and lifestyle, the more they will become a habit and the easier those changes will be to maintain.

Chapter 6

Paleo Diet Recipes for Diabetics

Now that you have a better understanding of the paleo diet and which foods are and are not included, you're ready to give it a try for yourself! In this chapter, you'll find a collection of delicious paleo recipes for breakfast, lunch, dinner, snacks, and dessert.

Recipes Included in this book

1	Blueberry Coconut Smoothie	2	Coco-Vanilla Chia Pudding
3	Tomato Basil Omelet	4	Spinach and Mushroom Omelet
5	Spiced Apple Walnut Muffins	6	Cinnamon Banana Pancakes
7	Ham and Red Pepper Frittata	8	Raspberry Kale Smoothie
9	Pumpkin Pie Pancakes	10	Pumpkin Pecan Muffins
11	Sweet Potato Breakfast Skillet	12	Vegetable Egg White Omelet
13	Strawberry Ginger Beet Smoothie	14	Cinnamon Coconut Flour Waffles
15	Triple Berry Smoothie	16	Thai Cocunut Vegetable Curry
17	Mixed Vegetable Frittata	18	Herb-Roasted Pork Tenderloin
19	Sweet Apple Pancakes	20	Balsamic Grilled Salmon
21	Blueberry Muffins	22	Veggie-Stuffed Salmon
23	Cinnamon Roasted Nuts	24	Slow Cooker Pulled Pork
25	Curried Butternut Squash Soup	26	Baked Beet Chips
27	Avocado Egg Salad	28	Meatloaf with BBQ Sauce

29	Roasted Tomato Basil Soup	30	Seared Scallops with Herb Butter
31	Avocado Spinach Salad with Egg	32	Herb-Crusted Lamb Chops
33	Creamy Sweet Potato Soup	34	Zucchini Pasta and Meatballs
35	Apple Walnut Chicken Salad	36	Almond Butter Brownies
37	Hearty Beef and Vegetable Stew	38	Chicken Tikka Masala
39	Balsamic Strawberry Kale Salad	40	Coconut Almond Chia Pudding
41	Cream of Broccoli Soup	42	Slow Cooker Balsamic Roast Beef
43	Chopped Chicken and Mango Salad	44	Cajun Chicken and Veggies
45	Mushroom and Leek Soup	46	Easy Garlic Shrimp
47	Creamy Cucumber Dill Salad	48	Bacon-Wrapped Turkey Breast
49	Lamb and Root Vegetable Stew	50	Grilled Salmon with Mango Sauce
51	Mango Walnut Salad with Pecans	52	Lemon Chicken with Broccoli
53	Easy Chicken and Vegetable Soup	54	Maple Walnut Trail Mix
55	Spiced Pumpkin Soup	56	Cilantro Lime Chicken
57	Rosemary Roasted Chicken	58	Curry Grilled Pork Chops
59	Baked Cinnamon Apple Chips	60	Lemon Blueberry Cupcakes
61	Avocado Deviled Eggs	62	Chocolate Chia Pudding
63	Sesame Kale Chips	64	Grilled Balsamic Peaches

Part 1

Breakfast Recipes

Blueberry Coconut Smoothie

Nutrition Facts (Per Serving): Calories: 59, Carbs: 7g, Fat: 1g, Protein: 6g

Servings: 1

Ingredients:

- 1 cup frozen blueberries
- ½ small frozen banana, sliced
- 1 cup unsweetened coconut milk
- ¼ cup canned coconut milk
- 1 teaspoon fresh lemon juice
- Ice cubes (optional)

Instructions:

1. Combine the blueberries and coconut milk in a blender.
2. Pulse the mixture several times to chop.
3. Add the remaining ingredients.
4. Blend on high speed for 30 to 60 seconds until smooth.
5. Pour the smoothie into a glass and enjoy right away.

Tomato Basil Omelet

Nutrition Facts (Per Serving): Calories: 274, Carbs: 5g, Fat: 21g, Protein: 18g

Servings: 1

Ingredients:

- 1 teaspoon olive oil, divided
- 1 small tomato, chopped
- ¼ cup diced yellow onion
- 1 clove minced garlic

- 2 large eggs, whisked
- 1 tablespoon chopped chives
- Salt and pepper
- 1 tablespoon fresh chopped basil

Instructions:

1. Heat ½ teaspoon of olive oil in a small skillet over medium heat.
2. Add the tomato, onions, and garlic – sauté for 3 to 4 minutes until tender.
3. Spoon the vegetables off into a bowl and reheat the skillet with the remaining oil.
4. Whisk together the eggs, chives, salt and pepper.
5. Pour the egg mixture into the skillet and let it cook for 1 minute.
6. Tilt the pan to spread the uncooked egg and cook until almost set.
7. Spoon the vegetable mixture over half the omelet and sprinkle with basil.
8. Fold the omelet over and cook until the egg is set.

Spiced Apple Walnut Muffins

Nutrition Facts (Per Serving): Calories: 180, Carbs: 28g, Fat: 6g, Protein: 4g

Servings: 1

Ingredients:

- 1 ¼ cups almond flour
- 3 tablespoons coconut flour
- 2 ½ teaspoons ground cinnamon
- ½ teaspoon baking soda
- ½ teaspoon ground nutmeg
- ¼ teaspoon salt
- 2 large eggs, whisked
- 1/3 cup melted coconut oil
- ¼ cup maple syrup

- 1 tablespoon vanilla extract
- ½ cup diced apples
- ¼ cup chopped walnuts

Instructions:

1. Preheat the oven to 350°F and line 8 cups of a regular muffin pan with paper liners.
2. Combine the almond flour, coconut flour, cinnamon, baking soda, nutmeg and salt in a mixing bowl.
3. In a separate bowl, whisk together the eggs, coconut oil, maple syrup, and vanilla extract until smooth.
4. Stir the dry ingredients into the wet until just combined.
5. Fold in the chopped apples and walnuts then divide the batter evenly among the muffin cups.
6. Bake for 22 to 25 minutes until a knife inserted in the center comes out clean.
7. Cool the muffins for 5 minutes in the pan then remove to a wire cooling rack.

Ham and Red Pepper Frittata

Nutrition Facts (Per Serving): Calories: 163, Carbs: 10g, Fat: 0g, Protein: 19g

Servings: 4

Ingredients:

- 8 large eggs, whisked
- ½ cup unsweetened almond milk
- 1 tablespoon olive oil
- 2 small red bell peppers, cored and chopped
- 1 small red onion, chopped
- 2 cloves minced garlic
- Salt and pepper
- 1 cup diced ham

Instructions:

1. Preheat the oven to 400°F.
2. Whisk together the eggs and almond milk in a bowl then set aside.
3. Heat the oil in a large oven-proof skillet over medium-high heat then add the peppers, onion, and garlic.
4. Cook for 5 to 6 minutes until the vegetables are just tender.
5. Season with salt and pepper to taste.
6. Pour the egg mixture into the skillet and sprinkle in the ham.
7. Let cook for 3 to 4 minutes until the egg begins to set around the edges.
8. Transfer the skillet to the preheated oven and cook for 10 minutes or so until the center is almost set.
9. Remove from the oven and let sit for 5 minutes before slicing to serve.

Pumpkin Protein Pancakes

Nutrition Facts (Per Serving): Calories: 378, Carbs: 32g, Fat: 13g, Protein: 33g

Servings: 5

Ingredients:

- ½ cup pumpkin (122 grams)
- 2 tablespoons coconut flour
- 2 tablespoons tapioca flour
- 1 serving Vital Proteins Collagen Peptides (2 scoops/20 grams)
- ½ teaspoon baking soda
- 1 teaspoon pumpkin pie spice
- Avocado oil, for greasing

Instructions:

1. Add pumpkin and eggs to a medium sized mixing bowl. Whisk until combined.

2. Add the dry ingredients and whisk again until well combined. Let sit for 5 minutes.
3. Melt avocado oil in a large sauté pan or griddle over medium heat.
4. Add about 1/4 cup of batter to the pan, forming pancakes. Cook for 2-3 minutes, then flip over and cook for another 2-3 minutes until fluffy and cooked through.
5. Repeat with remaining batter.
6. Serve with your favorite toppings and enjoy!

Strawberry Ginger Beet Smoothie

Nutrition Facts (Per Serving): Calories: 219, Carbs: 34g, Fat: 6g, Protein: 9g

Servings: 2

Ingredients:

- 1 cup frozen strawberries
- 1 cup chopped raw beets
- 1 banana
- I cup dairy free milk
- Juice of ½ lemon
- ½ teaspoon cinnamon
- ½ - 1 inch fresh ginger, peeled (start with ½ inch, you can always add more if you want it spicier)
- 1 tablespoon flax seeds
- 1 tablespoon hulled hemp seed
- 1 teaspoon fresh grated ginger

Instructions:

1. Combine the strawberries and beets in a blender.
2. Pulse the mixture several times to chop.
3. Add the remaining ingredients.
4. Blend on high speed for 30 to 60 seconds until smooth.

5. Pour the smoothie into a glass and enjoy right away.

Sweet Potato Breakfast Skillet

Nutrition Facts (Per Serving): Calories: 174, Carbs: 2g, Fat: 15g, Protein: 7g

Servings: 3

Ingredients:

- 2 tablespoon olive oil
- 2 large sweet potatoes, peeled and diced
- 3 pieces uncured bacon
- 3 large eggs
- ¼ cup white onion, diced
- 2 tablespoons green onion, chopped
- Salt and pepper to taste

Instructions:

1. Preheat oven to 400 F and prepare a baking sheet with parchment paper. Toss the cubed sweet potatoes in a bowl with 1 tablespoon of olive oil until well coated.
2. Transfer the sweet potatoes to the baking sheet and bake for 20-30 minutes OR you can toss them in the air fryer at 400F for 10 minutes.
3. In a large cast iron skillet over medium heat, cook the bacon and onion in 1 tablespoon olive oil until bacon is thoroughly cooked and onion is tender.
4. Once the sweet potatoes are done, add them to skillet with the onion and bacon.
5. Continue to cook for an additional 1-2 minutes and season with salt and pepper.
6. Turn the oven broiler to high. Create three wells in the sweet potatoes and crack an egg in each.
7. Place the skillet into the broil heated oven and cook for 2-3 minutes.
8. Top with green onion and more seasoning if desired.

Coco-Vanilla Chia Pudding

Nutrition Facts (Per Serving): Calories: 298, Carbs: 5g, Fat: 6g, Protein: 4g

Servings: 4

Ingredients:

- 1 (13.5-ounce) can coconut milk
- ¼ cup unsweetened almond milk
- 2 to 3 tablespoons honey
- 2 teaspoons vanilla extract
- ¼ cup chia seeds

Instructions:

1. Whisk together the coconut milk, almond milk, honey, and vanilla in a bowl.
2. Add the chia seeds and whisk until thoroughly combined.
3. Cover and chill overnight.
4. Spoon into bowls and top with fresh fruit and nuts to serve.

Spinach and Mushroom Omelet

Nutrition Facts (Per Serving): Calories: 278, Carbs: 5.4g, Fat: 25g, Protein: 22g

Servings: 1

Ingredients:

- 1 teaspoon olive oil, divided
- ½ cup diced mushrooms
- ¼ cup diced yellow onion
- 1 clove minced garlic

- ¼ cup frozen spinach, thawed and drained
- 2 large eggs, whisked
- Salt and pepper

Instructions:

1. Heat ½ teaspoon of olive oil in a small skillet over medium heat.
2. Add the mushrooms, onions, and garlic – sauté for 3 to 4 minutes until tender.
3. Stir in the spinach and cook for 30 seconds or until just heated through.
4. Spoon the vegetables off into a bowl and reheat the skillet with the remaining oil.
5. Whisk together the eggs, salt and pepper.
6. Pour the egg mixture into the skillet and let it cook for 1 minute.
7. Tilt the pan to spread the uncooked egg and cook until almost set.
8. Spoon the vegetable mixture over half the omelet then fold the omelet over and cook until the egg is set.

Raspberry Kale Smoothie

Nutrition Facts (Per Serving): Calories: 216, Carbs: 37g, Fat: 1g, Protein: 4g

Servings: 1

Ingredients:

- 1 cup frozen raspberries
- 1 cup fresh chopped kale
- 1 cup unsweetened apple juice
- ½ cup ice cubes
- 1 tablespoon fresh lemon juice
- 1 teaspoon honey

Instructions:

1. Combine the raspberries, kale and apple juice in a blender.

2. Pulse the mixture several times to chop.
3. Add the remaining ingredients.
4. Blend on high speed for 30 to 60 seconds until smooth.
5. Pour the smoothie into a glass and enjoy right away.

Light & Fluffy Banana Protein Pancake

Nutrition Facts (Per Serving): Calories: 198, Carbs: 18g, Fat: 5g, Protein: 22g

Servings: 8

Ingredients:

- 2 20g each scoops vanilla protein powder
- 1 large very ripe banana
- 1/8 teaspoon cinnamon
- ¼ teaspoon baking powder
- ¼ teaspoon salt
- 2 eggs

Instructions:

1. In two clean bowls, separate the eggs carefully so none of the yolk gets into the egg whites.
2. Beat the egg whites on high for 2 minutes until they form soft peaks. (It is important that your bowl or beaters don't have any oil, fat or yolks on them, or the egg whites won't form peaks. Soft peaks are defined as barely holding their shape. The peaks flop over immediately when the beaters are lifted.)
3. Add the remaining ingredients to the egg yolks and beat until smooth.
4. Gently fold 1/3 of the egg white mixture into the banana mixture until roughly combined.
5. Fold half of the remaining eggs whites into the mixture and finally the last portion until everything is well combined.
6. Heat a skillet over low heat. Scoop 1/4 c. of the mixture onto the skillet and cook for 60-90 seconds on each side.

7. Serve immediately.

Creamy Avocado Walnut Smoothie

Nutrition Facts (Per Serving): Calories: 370, Carbs: 10g, Fat: 29g, Protein: 9g

Servings: 1

Ingredients:

- 1 large frozen banana, sliced
- ½ ripe avocado, chopped
- 1 cup unsweetened almond milk
- ½ cup ice cubes
- 2 tablespoons chopped walnuts
- Pinch ground cinnamon

Instructions:

1. Combine the banana, avocado, and almond milk in a blender.
2. Pulse the mixture several times to chop.
3. Add the remaining ingredients.
4. Blend on high speed for 30 to 60 seconds until smooth.
5. Pour the smoothie into a glass and enjoy right away.

Vegetable Egg White Omelet

Nutritional Facts (Per Serving): Calories: 303, Carbs: 21g, Fat: 16g, Protein: 23g

Servings: 1

Ingredients:

- 1 teaspoon olive oil, divided

- 1 small tomato, chopped
- ¼ cup diced mushrooms
- ¼ cup diced yellow onion
- 2 tablespoons diced red pepper
- 1 clove minced garlic
- 3 large egg whites, whisked
- 1 tablespoon chopped chives
- Salt and pepper

Instructions:

1. Heat ½ teaspoon of olive oil in a small skillet over medium heat.
2. Add the vegetables and garlic – sauté for 3 to 4 minutes until tender.
3. Spoon the vegetables off into a bowl and reheat the skillet with the remaining oil.
4. Whisk together the eggs, chives, salt and pepper.
5. Pour the egg mixture into the skillet and let it cook for 1 minute.
6. Tilt the pan to spread the uncooked egg and cook until almost set.
7. Spoon the vegetable mixture over half the omelet.
8. Fold the omelet over and cook until the egg is set.

Cinnamon Coconut Flour Waffles

Nutritional Facts (Per Serving): Calories: 131, Carbs: 9g, Fat: 3g, Protein: 7g

Servings: 1

Ingredients:

- 1 whole egg (or 2 egg whites)
- 2 tablespoons coconut flour
- ¼ teaspoon baking powder
- ½ teaspoon ground cinnamon
- 3 tablespoons of dairy free milk (like almond, coconut etc.)

Instructions:

1. Mix everything together in a small bowl until no lumps remain. The end batter should be thick but easy to spread.
2. Divide the batter between two plates on a waffle iron and cook according to your waffle iron instructions.
3. Top with your favorite waffle toppings and enjoy!

Triple Berry Smoothie

Nutrition Facts (Per Serving): Calories: 140, Carbs: 27g, Fat: 1g, Protein: 5g

Servings: 1

Ingredients:

- ½ cup strawberries, fresh or frozen
- ½ cup frozen raspberries, fresh or frozen
- ¼ cup frozen blueberries, fresh or frozen
- ½ cup nonfat milk
- 2-3 ice cubes

Instructions:

1. Combine the berries and almond milk in a blender.
2. Pulse the mixture several times to chop.
3. Add the remaining ingredients.
4. Blend on high speed for 30 to 60 seconds until smooth.
5. Pour the smoothie into a glass and enjoy right away.

Mixed Vegetable Frittata

Nutrition Facts (Per Serving): Calories: 195, Carbs: 10g, Fat: 9g, Protein: 12g

Servings: 4

Ingredients:

- 8 large eggs, whisked
- ½ cup unsweetened almond milk
- 1 tablespoon olive oil
- 1 medium onion, chopped
- 1 small bell pepper, cored and chopped
- ½ cup diced broccoli florets
- ½ cup diced tomatoes
- 2 cloves minced garlic
- Salt and pepper

Instructions:

1. Preheat the oven to 400°F.
2. Whisk together the eggs and almond milk in a bowl then set aside.
3. Heat the oil in a large oven-proof skillet over medium-high heat.
4. Add the onion, peppers, broccoli, tomato, and garlic.
5. Cook for 5 to 6 minutes until the vegetables are just tender.
6. Season with salt and pepper to taste.
7. Pour the egg mixture into the skillet and let cook for 3 to 4 minutes until the egg begins to set around the edges.
8. Transfer the skillet to the preheated oven and cook for 10 minutes or so until the center is almost set.
9. Remove from the oven and let sit for 5 minutes before slicing to serve.

Chocolate Almond Butter Smoothie

Nutrition Facts: Calories: 189, Carbs: 10g, Fat: 17g, Protein: 5g

Servings: 1

Ingredients:

- Cacao powder raw chocolate powder certified organic by Navitas
- 1 cup unsweetened almond milk
- 1 cup ice cubes
- 2 tablespoons almond butter
- 4g Chia seeds
- 7 drops stevia liquid
- ½ avocado

Instructions:

1. Combine all ingredients in the blender, except avocado. You can use a stick blender for this, but start on low so the ingredients don't spill over!
2. Add avocado and blend
3. Serve cold!

Part 2

Lunch Recipes

Curried Butternut Squash Soup

Nutrition Facts (Per Serving): Calories: 275, Carbs: 32g, Fat: 13g, Protein: 7g

Servings: 4

Ingredients:

- 2 tablespoons olive oil, divided
- 6 cups chopped butternut squash
- 1 large sweet onion, chopped
- 1 tablespoon fresh grated ginger
- 1 tablespoon minced garlic
- 2 teaspoons curry powder
- ¼ teaspoon ground mustard powder
- Salt and pepper to taste
- 4 cups chicken stock (low sodium)

Instructions:

1. Heat 1 tablespoon oil in a large saucepan over medium heat.
2. Add the butternut squash and sauté for 6 to 8 minutes until browned.
3. Spoon the squash into a bowl and reheat the skillet with the remaining oil.
4. Add the onions, curry powder, garlic, ginger, mustard powder, salt and pepper.
5. Cook for 4 to 6 minutes until the onions are translucent.
6. Add the squash back to the pot along with the chicken stock.
7. Bring to a boil then reduce heat and simmer, covered, for 45 minutes.
8. Turn off the heat and puree the soup using an immersion blender until smooth.
9. Spoon into bowls and serve hot.

Avocado Egg Salad

Nutrition Facts (Per Serving): Calories: 229, Carbs: 7g, Fat: 18g, Protein: 12g

Servings: 4

Ingredients:

- 6 large hardboiled eggs, peeled and chopped
- 1 large ripe avocado, pitted and diced
- 2 tablespoons fresh lemon juice
- 6 slices cooked bacon, crumbled
- 2 green onions, sliced thin
- Paprika to taste

Instructions:

1. Combine the avocado and hardboiled egg in a bowl.
2. Mash the two ingredients together using a fork.
3. Stir in the lemon juice and salt then toss in the bacon and green onion.
4. Season with paprika to taste then chill until ready to serve.

Roasted Tomato Basil Soup

Nutrition Facts (Per Serving): Calories: 90, Carbs: 18g, Fat: 5g, Protein: 4g

Servings: 4

Ingredients:

- 4 large vine-ripened tomatoes, sliced
- 1 large sweet onion, sliced
- 6 cloves fresh garlic, sliced

- Olive oil, as needed
- Salt and pepper
- 2 cups vegetable broth
- 2 tablespoons tomato paste
- ¼ cup fresh chopped basil

Instructions:

1. Preheat the oven to 350°F.
2. Spread the tomatoes, onions, and garlic on a foil-lined baking sheet and drizzle with oil.
3. Season with salt and pepper then toss gently.
4. Roast for 40 minutes, stirring once halfway through, until very tender.
5. Heat the vegetable stock in a large saucepan over medium heat.
6. Whisk in the tomato paste and basil then add the roasted vegetables.
7. Bring to a boil then reduce heat and simmer, covered, for 10 minutes.
8. Turn off the heat and puree the soup using an immersion blender until smooth.
9. Spoon into bowls and serve hot.

Avocado Spinach Salad with Egg

Nutrition Facts (Per Serving): Calories: 230, Carbs: 9g, Fat: 18g, Protein: 13g

Servings: 4

Ingredients:

- 5 cups fresh baby spinach
- 1 cup thinly sliced mushrooms
- ½ small red onion, sliced thin
- 1 large avocado, pitted and sliced thin
- 4 hardboiled eggs, peeled and sliced

Instructions:

1. Combine the spinach, mushrooms, and red onion in a large salad bowl.
2. Toss well then divide among four salad plates.
3. Top each salad with slices of avocado and hardboiled egg.
4. Drizzle with your favorite paleo dressing to serve.

Apple Walnut Chicken Salad

Nutrition Facts (Per Serving): Calories: 400, Carbs: 23g, Fat: 21g, Protein: 34g

Servings: 4

Ingredients:

- 2 tablespoons olive oil
- 1 tablespoon fresh lemon juice
- 2 tablespoons fresh chopped parsley
- 2 cloves minced garlic
- Salt and pepper to taste
- 2 cups cooked chicken breast, chopped
- 1 small ripe avocado, pitted and chopped
- 1 small green apple, peeled and diced
- ¼ cup diced celery
- ¼ cup sliced green onion
- ¼ cup chopped walnuts

Instructions:

1. Whisk together the olive oil, lemon juice, parsley, garlic, salt and pepper in a mixing bowl.
2. Toss in the cooked chicken, avocado, apple, celery, green onion, and walnuts until evenly coated.
3. Serve on a bed of lettuce.

Hearty Beef and Vegetable Stew

Nutrition Facts (Per Serving): Calories: 385, Carbs: 21g, Fat: 19g, Protein: 44g

Servings: 1

Ingredients:

- 1 tablespoon olive oil
- 2 medium sweet potatoes, peeled and chopped
- 2 large carrots, peeled and sliced
- 1 large yellow onion, chopped
- 1 cup sliced celery
- 1 pound beef stew meat, chopped
- 2 (14-ounce) cans diced tomatoes
- 4 cups beef stock (low sodium)
- 1 teaspoon fresh chopped rosemary
- ½ teaspoon fresh chopped thyme
- Salt and pepper

Instructions:

1. Heat the oil in a large saucepan over medium-high heat.
2. Add the sweet potatoes, carrots, onion, and celery and cook for 4 to 5 minutes until lightly browned.
3. Stir in the beef along with the tomatoes, stock, and seasonings.
4. Bring the mixture to a boil then reduce heat and simmer, covered, for one hour – stir every 15 minutes.
5. Uncover the pot and simmer for another 45 minutes then serve hot.

Cream of Broccoli Soup

Nutrition Facts (Per Serving): Calories: 210, Carbs: 19g, Fat: 13g, Protein: 4g

Servings: 4

Ingredients:

- 1 tablespoon olive oil
- 1 medium white onion, chopped
- 2 cloves minced garlic
- 3 cups chicken broth (low sodium)
- 1 pound fresh chopped broccoli
- 1 medium leek, sliced (white and light green parts only)
- Salt and pepper
- 1 cup canned coconut milk

Instructions:

1. Heat the oil in a large saucepan over medium-high heat.
2. Add the onions and cook for 4 to 5 minutes until translucent.
3. Stir in the garlic and cook for 1 minute more.
4. Add the broth, broccoli, and leeks then season with salt and pepper.
5. Bring to a boil then reduce heat and simmer for 20 minutes until the broccoli is very tender.
6. Turn off the heat and puree the soup using an immersion blender.
7. Stir in the coconut milk and adjust seasoning to taste. Serve hot.

Chopped Chicken and Mango Salad

Nutrition Facts (Per Serving): Calories: 444, Carbs: 18g, Fat: 29g, Protein: 27g

Servings: 1

Ingredients:

- 1 tablespoon olive oil
- 1 pound boneless skinless chicken breast, chopped
- 1 teaspoon chili powder

- Salt and pepper
- ½ cup olive oil mayonnaise
- 1 ½ tablespoons fresh lime juice
- 3 cloves minced garlic
- ½ red pepper, cored and diced
- ¼ cup diced red onion
- 1 ripe mango, peeled and diced

Instructions:

1. Heat the oil in a large skillet over medium-high heat.
2. Add the chicken and season with chili powder, salt and pepper.
3. Sauté the chicken until evenly browned and cooked through then remove to a bowl and let cool.
4. Combine the mayonnaise, lime juice, and garlic in a mixing bowl.
5. Whisk well then toss in the chopped chicken, bell pepper, red onion, and mango.
6. Chill until ready to serve then serve over a bed of lettuce.

Mushroom and Leek Soup

Nutrition Facts (Per Serving): Calories: 180, Carbs: 17g, Fat: 9g, Protein: 5g

Servings: 4

Ingredients:

- 1 tablespoon olive oil
- 1 large leek, sliced thin (white and light green parts only)
- 1 ½ pounds fresh sliced mushrooms
- 1 small white onion, chopped
- 3 cloves minced garlic
- 2 cups vegetable broth (divided)
- 2 tablespoons arrowroot powder

- ¼ cup canned coconut milk
- 1 tablespoon fresh chopped thyme
- 1 tablespoon fresh chopped rosemary
- Salt and pepper, to taste

Instructions:

1. Heat the oil in a large saucepan over medium heat.
2. Add the leeks and cook for 4 to 5 minutes until just browned.
3. Stir in the mushrooms, onion, and garlic and cook for 6 to 8 minutes until tender.
4. Pour in 2 tablespoons of the vegetable broth and scrape up the browned bits from the bottom of the pan.
5. Stir in the arrowroot powder then stir in the coconut milk and the rest of the broth.
6. Bring the mixture to a simmer then stir in the herbs, salt, and pepper.
7. Simmer the soup, covered, for 15 to 20 minutes then serve hot.

Creamy Cucumber Dill Salad

Nutrition Facts (Per Serving): Calories: 80, Carbs: 12g, Fat: 5g, Protein: 2g

Servings: 4

Ingredients:

- 2 large seedless cucumbers
- 1 small red onion, sliced thin
- ¼ cup canned coconut milk
- 2 tablespoons fresh chopped dill
- 1 tablespoon honey
- Salt and pepper to taste

Instructions:

1. Slice the cucumbers very thin and place them in a large bowl.

2. Add the sliced red onion and set aside.
3. Whisk together the coconut milk, dill, honey, salt, and pepper in a separate bowl.
4. Toss the dressing with the cucumber and onions to coat.
5. Chill the salad until ready to serve.

Lamb and Root Vegetable Stew

Nutrition Facts (Per Serving): Calories: 355, Carbs: 22g, Fat: 19g, Protein: 25g

Servings: 1

Ingredients:

- 1 tablespoon coconut oil
- 2 large carrots, peeled and sliced
- 2 medium turnips, peeled and sliced
- 1 large parsnip, peeled and sliced
- 1 large sweet potato, peeled and chopped
- 1 large yellow onion, chopped
- 1 pound lamb shank, chopped
- 2 (14-ounce) cans diced tomatoes
- 4 cups beef stock (low sodium)
- 1 teaspoon fresh chopped rosemary
- ½ teaspoon fresh chopped thyme
- Salt and pepper

Instructions:

1. Heat the oil in a large saucepan over medium-high heat.
2. Add the vegetables and cook for 4 to 5 minutes until lightly browned.
3. Stir in the lamb along with the tomatoes, stock, and seasonings.
4. Bring the mixture to a boil then reduce heat and simmer, covered, for one hour – stir every 15 minutes.

5. Uncover the pot and simmer for another 45 minutes then serve hot.

Easy Chicken and Vegetable Soup

Nutrition Facts (Per Serving): Calories: 157, Carbs: 24g, Fat: 4g, Protein: 18g

Servings: 6

Ingredients:

- 1 tablespoon olive oil
- 2 cups cooked chicken breast, chopped
- 1 medium yellow onion, chopped
- 1 small leek, sliced thin (white and light green parts only)
- 8 cups low sodium chicken stock
- 2 large carrots, peeled and sliced
- 1 medium zucchini, sliced
- 1 large stalk celery, sliced
- 1 red pepper, diced
- 1 cup diced tomatoes
- ¼ cup fresh chopped parsley
- 1 teaspoon fresh chopped thyme
- ½ teaspoon fresh chopped tarragon
- Salt and pepper

Instructions:

1. Heat the oil in a large stockpot over medium heat.
2. Add the chicken, onions, and leeks and cook for 4 to 5 minutes.
3. Stir in the remaining ingredients and bring to a boil.
4. Reduce heat and simmer for 20 minutes until the vegetables are tender and the chicken heated through.
5. Season with salt and pepper to taste and serve hot.

Spiced Pumpkin Soup

Nutrition Facts (Per Serving): Calories: 164, Carbs: 23g, Fat: 5g, Protein: 10g

Servings: 6

Ingredients:

- 1 tablespoon butter
- 1 cup onion, chopped
- 3 tablespoons coconut flour
- ½ teaspoon curry powder
- ¼ teaspoon cumin
- ¼ teaspoon ground nutmeg
- 2 garlic cloves, crushed
- 1 cup peeled and cubed sweet potato
- ¼ teaspoon salt
- 2 14oz. cans of low sodium chicken broth
- 1 15oz. can of pumpkin
- 1 cup 1% milk
- 1 tablespoon fresh lime juice

Instructions:

1. Heat 1 tablespoon oil in a large saucepan over medium heat.
2. Melt butter in a Dutch oven or large saucepan over medium-high heat.
3. Saute onion for 3-4 minutes then add flour, curry, garlic, cumin and nutmeg and sauté for 1 minute.
4. Add sweet potato, salt, chicken broth and pumpkin and bring to a boil. Reduce heat to medium-low and simmer, partially covered for about 20-25 minutes or until sweet potatoes are cooked through and softened.
5. Remove from heat and let stand for 10 minutes to cool

6. Place half of the pumpkin mixture in a blender and process until smooth.
7. Using a strainer, pour soup back into pan. Repeat with the rest of the soup
8. Raise heat to medium then stir in milk and cook for 5 minutes or until soup is heated through
9. Remove from heat and add lime juice

Part 3

Dinner Recipes

Rosemary Roasted Chicken

Nutrition Facts (Per Serving): Calories: 183, Carbs: 3g, Fat: 8g, Protein: 28g

Servings: 4

Ingredients:

- 2 to 3 pounds bone-in chicken drumsticks and thighs
- 2 tablespoons olive oil
- Salt and pepper
- 1 large yellow onion, quartered
- 1 large sweet potato, chopped coarsely
- 1 cup broccoli florets
- 1 cup cauliflower florets
- 1 cup baby carrots
- 1 red pepper, cored and chopped
- 1 green pepper, cored and chopped
- 1 tablespoon fresh chopped rosemary
- 1 teaspoon fresh chopped thyme
- ¼ cup chicken broth (low sodium)

Instructions:

1. Preheat the oven to 400°F.
2. Season the chicken with salt and pepper to taste.
3. Heat the oil in a large skillet over medium-high heat.
4. Add the chicken in batches and cook until evenly browned, turning as needed.
5. Combine the vegetables in a large bowl and toss to coat with oil, rosemary, and thyme.
6. Spread the vegetables in a large rectangular glass baking dish and arrange the chicken on top of it.
7. Drizzle with chicken broth then roast for 50 to 60 minutes until the chicken is cooked through and the vegetables tender.

Thai Coconut Vegetable Curry

Nutrition Facts (Per Serving): Calories: 187, Carbs: 24g, Fat: 7g, Protein: 7g

Servings: 4

Ingredients:

- 1 tablespoon coconut oil
- 1 medium yellow onion, chopped
- 1 tablespoon fresh grated ginger
- 1 tablespoon fresh minced garlic
- 1 cup sliced carrots
- 2 bell peppers, cored and chopped
- 2 tablespoons Thai curry paste
- 1 (14-ounce) can coconut milk (full fat)
- ½ cup vegetable broth
- 2 cups fresh chopped kale
- Salt, to taste

Instructions:

1. Heat the oil in a large skillet over medium heat.
2. Add the onion and cook until translucent – about 4 to 5 minutes.
3. Stir in the ginger and garlic and cook for another 30 seconds.
4. Add the carrots and bell peppers – cook for 4 to 5 minutes until tender, stirring occasionally.
5. Stir in the curry paste and cook for 2 minutes.
6. Add the coconut milk, vegetable broth, and kale then stir well.
7. Bring to a boil then reduce heat and simmer for 5 to 10 minutes until the vegetables are tender – stir as needed.
8. Season the curry with salt to taste and serve hot.

Herb-Roasted Pork Tenderloin

Nutrition Facts (Per Serving): Calories: 312, Carbs: 6g, Fat: 12g, Protein: 43g

Servings: 4

Ingredients:

- 1 (4-pound) boneless pork tenderloin
- Salt and pepper
- 2 tablespoons olive oil
- 4 shallots, sliced very thin
- 3 tablespoons Dijon mustard
- 2 tablespoons minced garlic
- 1 tablespoon fresh chopped rosemary
- 1 tablespoon fresh chopped thyme
- 1 tablespoon fresh chopped sage

Instructions:

1. Preheat the oven to 350°F.
2. Use a paper towel to pat the pork tenderloin dry then season generously with salt and pepper.
3. Heat the oil in a large skillet over medium-high heat then add the pork and brown on all sides.
4. Combine the sliced shallots, mustard, garlic, and herbs in a bowl.
5. Place the pork on a rack in a roasting pan and spread the herb mixture over it.
6. Roast the pork for 1 hour then keep cooking, checking every 5 minutes, until the internal temperature reads 140°F to 145°F.
7. Transfer the pork to a cutting board and let rest for 15 minutes before slicing.

Balsamic Grilled Salmon

Nutrition Facts (Per Serving): Calories: 284, Carbs: 6g, Fat: 12g, Protein: 37g

Servings: 4

Ingredients:

- Olive oil, as needed
- 3 tablespoons honey
- 2 tablespoons Dijon mustard
- 2 tablespoons balsamic vinegar
- ½ teaspoon salt
- ¼ teaspoon black pepper
- 4 (6-ounce) boneless salmon fillets
- Lemon wedges

Instructions:

1. Preheat a grill to medium-high heat and brush the grates with olive oil.
2. Whisk together the honey, Dijon mustard, balsamic vinegar, salt and pepper in a small bowl.
3. Brush the mixture over the salmon fillets and place them on the grill.
4. Cover the grill and cook for 2 to 3 minutes on each side until the flesh flakes easily with a fork.
5. Drizzle with extra glaze, if desired, and serve with lemon wedges.

Slow Cooker Pulled Pork

Nutrition Facts (Per Serving): Calories: 165, Carbs: 5g, Fat: 11g, Protein: 9g

Servings: 8

Ingredients:

- 4 pounds boneless pork shoulder
- ¼ cup smoked paprika
- 2 tablespoons chili powder
- 2 tablespoons ground cumin
- 1 tablespoon salt
- 1 tablespoon white pepper

- 1 to 2 cups barbecue sauce

Instructions:

1. Combine the paprika, chili powder, cumin, salt and pepper in a small bowl.
2. Rub the spice mixture into the pork shoulder on all sides.
3. Wrap the pork in two layers of plastic and chill for at least 4 hours.
4. Place the unwrapped pork shoulder in a slow cooker then pour in the water.
5. Cover and cook on low heat for 8 to 10 hours until the pork is very tender.
6. Transfer the pork to a cutting board and shred it with two forks.
7. Return the pork to the slow cooker with the juices and toss with your favorite paleo barbecue sauce.

Seared Scallops with Herb Butter

Nutrition Facts (Per Serving): Calories: 175, Carbs: 5g, Fat: 2g, Protein: 29g

Servings: 4

Ingredients:

- 1 tablespoon coconut oil
- 1 ¼ pounds large sea scallops, rinsed and patted dry
- Salt and pepper
- 3 tablespoons grass-fed butter, chopped
- 2 tablespoons fresh chopped herbs (your choice)
- 1 tablespoon fresh lemon juice

Instructions:

1. Heat the oil in a large skillet over medium-high heat.
2. Lightly season the scallops with salt and pepper then place them in the hot oil.
3. Sear for 2 to 3 minutes on one side until golden brown.
4. Carefully turn the scallops then add the butter and herbs to the skillet.

5. Cook for 2 to 3 minutes until the scallops are just cooked through.
6. Drizzle with lemon juice and serve hot.

Meatloaf with BBQ Sauce

Nutrition Facts (Per Serving): Calories: 161, Carbs: 14g, Fat: 2.8g, Protein: 18g

Servings: 1

Ingredients:

- 1 tablespoon olive oil
- 1 small yellow onion, chopped
- 3 cloves minced garlic
- 1 teaspoon fresh chopped oregano
- 1 teaspoon fresh chopped thyme
- Salt and pepper
- 1 pound lean ground beef
- 1 pound lean ground turkey breast
- 3 large eggs, whisked
- ½ cup almond flour
- ½ cup paleo barbecue sauce

Instructions:

1. Preheat the oven to 350°F.
2. Heat the oil in a small saucepan over medium heat until tender.
3. Stir in the onions, garlic, oregano, thyme, salt and pepper then remove from heat.
4. Place the ground beef and turkey in a large mixing bowl.
5. Add the eggs and almond flour, mixing it together by hand.
6. Work the vegetable mixture into the meat then shape it into a loaf and place it on a roasting pan.
7. Pour the barbecue sauce over the meatloaf.

8. Bake for 1 hour and 5 to 15 minutes until the internal temperature reaches 155°F.
9. Remove the meatloaf from the oven and let rest 10 minutes before serving.

Herb-Crusted Lamb Chops

Nutrition Facts (Per Serving): Calories: 237, Carbs: 5g, Fat: 13g, Protein: 23g

Servings: 4

Ingredients:

- 2 pounds bone-in lamb chops
- Salt and pepper
- 3 tablespoons olive oil
- 2 tablespoons minced garlic
- ¼ cup fresh chopped parsley
- ½ teaspoon fresh chopped rosemary
- ½ teaspoon fresh chopped thyme
- Coconut oil, as needed

Instructions:

1. Pat the lamb chops dry with paper towel and season with salt and pepper.
2. Whisk together the olive oil, garlic, parsley, rosemary, and thyme in a small bowl.
3. Arrange the lamb chops in a shallow dish and pour the marinade over them, turning to coat.
4. Cover and chill for 6 to 12 hours.
5. Take the lamb chops out of the refrigerator 30 minutes prior to cooking.
6. Heat some coconut oil in a large skillet over high heat.
7. Add the lamb chops and cook for 3 to 4 minutes on each side until seared.

Zucchini Pasta and Meatballs

Nutrition Facts (Per Serving): Calories: 373, Carbs: 30g, Fat: 17g, Protein: 27g

Servings: 1

Ingredients:

- 2 cups pasta sauce
- 3 large zucchini
- 1 pound lean ground beef
- 1 pound lean ground turkey
- 1 large egg, whisked
- ½ cup almond flour
- 2 ½ tablespoons coconut aminos
- 1 tablespoon Italian seasoning
- Salt to taste

Instructions:

1. Preheat the oven to 400°F and line a baking sheet with foil.
2. Place the pasta sauce in a saucepan and warm over medium heat.
3. Use a vegetable peeler or mandolin to slice the zucchini into noodle-like strips or threads.
4. Set the zucchini noodles aside while you prepare the meatballs.
5. Combine the beef, turkey, egg, almond flour, coconut aminos, Italian seasoning and salt in a bowl, mixing by hand.
6. Shape the mixture into 1-inch balls and arrange them on the baking sheet.
7. Bake for 18 to 22 minutes until the meatballs are cooked through.
8. Heat some oil in a large skillet over medium heat.
9. Add the zucchini and cook until just heated through then serve with the meatballs and pasta sauce.

Chicken Tikka Masala

Nutrition Facts (Per Serving): Calories: 260, Carbs: 14g, Fat: 11g, Protein: 26g

Servings: 4

Ingredients:

- 1 tablespoon rapeseed oil
- 1 large onion, chopped
- 1 red pepper, finely chopped
- 2 skinless chicken breasts, cubes
- 2 tablespoon tikka paste
- 2-3 cloves of garlic, crushed
- 1 x 400g tin chopped tomatoes
- 2 tablespoon freshly chopped coriander plus 2 teaspoon to serve
- 2 tablespoon 0% fat Greek yogurt
- 1 medium yellow onion, chopped

Instructions:

1. Add the oil to a pan and add the onions and peppers. Cook for 5 minutes until soft and add the chicken breasts and cook for 3 minutes.
2. Add the tikka paste and stir for 1-2 minutes until the chicken is evenly coated.
3. Add the garlic and tomatoes, mix again and bring to a gentle boil then cover and simmer gently for 6-8 minutes.
4. Add the coriander, stir well then remove from the heat.
5. Stir in the yogurt, sprinkle with the remaining coriander and serve immediately.

Slow Cooker Balsamic Roast Beef

Nutrition Facts (Nutrition Facts): Calories: 225, Carbs: 6g, Fat: 5g, Protein: 36g

Servings: 4

Ingredients:

- 3 pounds boneless beef chuck roast
- Salt and pepper
- 2 tablespoons coconut oil
- 1 large yellow onion, sliced
- 1 tablespoon minced garlic
- 2 cups beef stock
- ½ cup balsamic vinegar
- 2 tablespoons fresh chopped rosemary
- 3 large sweet potatoes, chopped
- 4 medium carrots, peeled and sliced

Instructions:

1. Season the chuck roast with salt and pepper.
2. Heat the oil in a large skillet over medium-high heat.
3. Add the roast and cook until it is browned on all sides, about 2 to 3 minutes per side.
4. Place the roast in a slow cooker and add the onion and garlic.
5. Drizzle in the beef stock and balsamic vinegar then sprinkle with rosemary.
6. Cover and cook on low heat for 6 hours.
7. Add the sweet potatoes and carrots then cook, covered, on high for 3 hours until the meat is very tender.
8. Remove the roast to a cutting board and cover loosely with foil.
9. Use a slotted spoon to remove the vegetables to a bowl then pour the cooking liquid into a saucepan.

10. Bring the liquid to a slow boil and simmer until it thickens.
11. Slice the roast and serve with the vegetables, drizzled in sauce.

Cajun Chicken and Veggies

Nutrition Facts (Per Serving): Calories: 244, Carbs: 8g, Fat: 15g, Protein: 22g

Servings: 4

Ingredients:

- Olive oil, as needed
- 3 pounds bone-in chicken thighs
- 1 tablespoon paprika
- 2 teaspoons garlic powder
- 2 teaspoons salt
- 1 ½ teaspoons dried oregano
- 1 ½ teaspoons dried thyme
- 1 teaspoon onion powder
- 1 teaspoon black pepper
- ½ teaspoon cayenne
- 2 pounds sweet potatoes, chopped
- 1 red pepper, cored and chopped
- 1 small red onion, chopped

Instructions:

1. Rub the olive oil into the chicken and place it on a rimmed baking sheet.
2. Combine the spices in a small bowl then rub the mixture into both sides of the chicken.
3. Place the sweet potatoes in a large bowl and drizzle with oil then toss with some of the spice mixture.
4. Spread the sweet potatoes on the baking sheet around the chicken and roast for 30 minutes.

5. Sprinkle on the red pepper and onions and roast for another 10 to 15 minutes until the chicken is cooked through.
6. Serve the chicken hot with the roasted vegetables.

Easy Garlic Shrimp

Nutrition Facts (Per Serving): Calories: 224, Carbs: 2g, Fat: 10g, Protein: 32g

Servings: 4

Ingredients:

- 3 tablespoons olive oil
- 2 tablespoons minced garlic
- 1 ¼ pound large uncooked shrimp, peeled and deveined
- 1 teaspoon salt
- ¼ teaspoon pepper
- Paprika, as needed

Instructions:

1. Heat the oil in a large skillet over medium-low heat.
2. Add the garlic and cook for 2 to 3 minutes until softened and fragrant.
3. Place the shrimp in the skillet in a single layer then increase the heat to medium-high.
4. Season the shrimp with salt and pepper as well as a pinch of paprika.
5. Cook the shrimp for 2 to 3 minutes until the bottom half turns pink.
6. Flip the shrimp and cook for another minute or two until just opaque.

Bacon-Wrapped Turkey Breast

Nutrition Facts (Per Serving): Calories: 285, Carbs: 3g, Fat: 17g, Protein: 29g

Servings: 6

Ingredients:

- 4 pounds boneless skinless turkey breast
- 10 to 12 slices uncooked bacon
- Salt and pepper
- 2 tablespoons olive oil

Instructions:

1. Preheat the oven to 400°F.
2. Cut the turkey breast into chunks then season with salt and pepper.
3. Wrap each piece of turkey in a slice of bacon.
4. Heat the oil in a large cast-iron skillet over medium-high heat.
5. Add the turkey to the skillet and cook for 2 minutes until the underside is browned.
6. Flip the turkey and transfer the skillet to the oven.
7. Cook for 10 to 15 minutes until the turkey is cooked through and the bacon is crispy. Serve hot.

Grilled Salmon with Mango Sauce

Nutrition Facts (Per Serving): Calories: 126, Carbs: 5g, Fat: 4g, Protein: 26g

Servings: 4

Ingredients:

- 4 (6-ounce) boneless salmon fillets
- Olive oil
- Salt and pepper
- 1 ripe mango, pitted and chopped
- ¼ cup canned coconut milk
- 2 tablespoons fresh chopped cilantro
- 1 teaspoon fresh lime juice

Instructions:

1. Preheat a grill to medium-high heat and brush the grates with olive oil.
2. Season the salmon fillets with salt and pepper then place them on the grill.
3. Cover the grill and cook for 2 to 3 minutes on each side until the flesh flakes easily with a fork.
4. While the salmon cooks, combine the remaining ingredients in a food processor or blender.
5. Blend until smooth then serve drizzled over the grilled salmon.

Lemon Chicken with Broccoli

Nutrition Facts (Per Serving): Calories: 175, Carbs: 10g, Fat: 8g, Protein: 18g

Servings: 4

Ingredients:

- 2 tablespoons olive oil
- 4 large boneless skinless chicken breasts
- Salt and pepper
- Italian seasoning, to taste
- 1 cup low-sodium chicken broth
- ¼ cup fresh lemon juice
- 1 tablespoon minced garlic
- 1 (10-ounce) bag frozen broccoli florets
- 1 large lemon, sliced

Instructions:

1. Heat the oil in a large skillet over medium heat.
2. Season the chicken with salt, pepper, and Italian seasoning then add it to the skillet.
3. Cook for 3 to 4 minutes until the underside is browned then turn the chicken and brown on the other side.
4. Remove the chicken to a plate and reheat the skillet.

5. Add the chicken broth, lemon juice, and garlic, stirring to scrape up any browned bits from the bottom of the pan.
6. Add the chicken to the skillet along with the lemon.
7. Simmer for 5 minutes, turning the chicken halfway through.
8. Add the broccoli and cook for 5 minutes or until it is bright green and tender-crisp.
9. Adjust seasoning to taste and serve hot.

Maple Country Style Pork Ribs

Nutrition Facts (Per Serving): Calories: 189, Carbs: 3g, Fat: 10g, Protein: 23g

Servings: 4

Ingredients:

- ¼ teaspoon ground allspice
- ¼ teaspoon ground cinnamon
- 2 pounds country-style pork ribs (to yield 16 ounces meat before cooking)
- ¼ cup onion, diced
- ¼ teaspoon ground allspice
- ½ teaspoon garlic powder
- 1 tablespoon sugar-free maple-flavored syrup
- 1 dash black pepper
- ¼ teaspoon ground ginger
- 1 tablespoon coconut aminos (soy-free seasoning sauce)

Instructions:

1. Combine all ingredients except the ribs in a medium bowl. Pour over the ribs.
2. If baking in the oven, place the ribs in a baking dish, cover with foil and bake for 60-90 minutes, or until internal temperature reaches 180 degrees.
3. If preparing in the crockpot, covet and cook on low for 7-9 hours

Cilantro Lime Chicken

Nutrition Facts (Per Serving): Calories: 81, Carbs: 3g, Fat: 2g, Protein: 8g

Servings: 4

Ingredients:

- ¼ cup olive oil
- ¼ cup fresh chopped cilantro
- 2 tablespoons lime juice
- 1 tablespoon minced garlic
- 1 teaspoon ground cumin
- ½ teaspoon red pepper flakes
- 2 pounds boneless chicken thighs
- Salt and pepper
- 2 tablespoons cooking oil

Instructions:

1. Whisk together the olive oil, cilantro, lime juice, garlic, cumin, and red pepper flakes in a bowl.
2. Place the chicken in a shallow dish and season with salt and pepper.
3. Pour the marinade over it, turning to coat, then cover and chill for up to 2 hours.
4. Preheat the oven to 375°F.
5. Melt the coconut oil in a large ovenproof skillet over medium-high heat.
6. Add the chicken and cook until browned on both sides, about 2 to 3 minutes.
7. Transfer the chicken to the oven and bake for 15 to 20 minutes until cooked through.
8. Sprinkle with cilantro and drizzle with lime juice to serve.

Curry Grilled Pork Chops

Nutrition Facts (Per Serving): Calories: 289, Carbs: 8g, Fat: 28g, Protein: 5g

Servings: 4

Ingredients:

- 4 bone-in pork chops, 1-inch thick
- Salt and pepper
- 1 tablespoon olive oil
- 1 ½ teaspoons curry powder

Instructions:

1. Preheat the grill to high heat and brush the grates with oil.
2. Season the pork chops with salt and pepper to taste then place them in a shallow dish.
3. Whisk together the olive oil and curry powder then pour over the pork chops, turning to coat.
4. Place the pork chops on the grill and cook for 3 to 4 minutes on each side until just cooked through.
5. Remove the pork chops to a cutting board and let rest 5 minutes before serving.

Part 4

Snacks & Desserts

Baked Cinnamon Apple Chips

Nutrition Facts (Per Serving): Calories: 110, Carbs: 25g, Fat: 1g, Protein: 1g

Servings: 2

Ingredients:

- 1 parchment paper
- 1 medium apple
- 1 teaspoon ground cinnamon

Instructions:

1. Preheat the oven to 225°F and line two baking sheets with parchment.
2. Slice the apples as thinly as possible and arrange them on the baking sheet in a single layer.
3. Sprinkle with cinnamon then bake for 1 hour.
4. Flip the apple slices and let them cook for another hour.
5. Turn off the oven and let the slices cool until crisp then store in an airtight container.

Avocado Deviled Eggs

Nutrition Facts (Per Serving): Calories: 345, Carbs: 3g, Fat: 25g, Protein: 26g

Servings: 1

Ingredients:

- 4 large hard boiled eggs
- 3 tablespoons avocado/guacamole
- ½ tablespoon sour cream
- ½ teaspoon lime juice
- ¼ teaspoon cayenne pepper
- ½ teaspoon black pepper
- ¼ teaspoon pink Himalayan salt

Instructions:

1. Cut 4 hard boiled eggs in half, creating 8 halves.
2. Scoop the yolks out of the whites into a bowl and set whites aside.
3. Mash up the avocado and add it to the yolks along with the sour cream, lime juice, cayenne, pepper and salt. Combine.
4. Scoop yolk mixture evenly into the center of the whites.
5. Garnish with jalapeno slice. Store in fridge and enjoy!

Chocolate Chia Pudding

Nutrition Facts (Per Serving): Calories: 165, Carbs: 11g, Fat: 13g, Protein: 5g

Servings: 4

Ingredients:

- 1 ½ cups unsweetened almond milk
- 8 pitted Medjool dates
- ¼ cup unsweetened cocoa powder
- ¼ cup chia seeds
- 1 teaspoon vanilla extract

Instructions:

1. Combine the almond milk, dates, cocoa powder, chia seeds, and vanilla extract in a blender.
2. Blend on high speed for 30 to 60 seconds, scraping down the sides as needed, until smooth and well combined.
3. Spoon into dessert cups and chill until ready to serve.

Sesame Kale Chips

Nutrition Facts (Per Serving): Calories: 91, Carbs: 12g, Fat: 4g, Protein: 4g

Servings: 4

Ingredients:

- 2 large bunches of fresh kale
- Sesame oil, as needed
- Salt, as needed
- Sesame seeds, as needed

Instructions:

1. Preheat the oven to 350°F and line two baking sheets with parchment.
2. Trim the stems from the kale and cut the leaves into 2-inch pieces then arrange them on the baking sheet in a single layer.
3. Drizzle with oil and sprinkle with salt then bake for 12 minutes.
4. Sprinkle with sesame seeds then store in an airtight container.

Almond Butter Brownies

Nutrition Facts (Per Serving): Calories: 282, Carbs: 26g, Fat: 20g, Protein: 5g

Servings: 8 to 10

Ingredients:

- 1 cup smooth almond butter
- 1/3 cup honey
- 1 large egg, whisked
- 2 tablespoons melted coconut oil

- 1 teaspoon vanilla extract
- 1/3 cup unsweetened cocoa powder
- ½ teaspoon baking soda

Instructions:

1. Preheat the oven to 325°F and grease a square baking pan.
2. Combine the almond butter, honey, egg, coconut oil, and vanilla extract in a mixing bowl.
3. Whisk until smooth and well combined.
4. Stir together the cocoa powder and baking soda in another bowl then stir the dry ingredients into the wet.
5. Spread the batter in the prepared pan and bake for 20 to 23 minutes until the brownies are set in the middle.
6. Cool the brownies completely before cutting to serve.

Cinnamon Roasted Nuts

Nutrition Facts (Per Serving): Calories: 231, Carbs: 18g, Fat: 13g, Protein: 8g

Servings: 6 to 8

Ingredients:

- 2 cups whole almonds
- 2 to 3 teaspoons olive oil
- 1 teaspoon ground cinnamon
- ½ teaspoon salt

Instructions:

1. Preheat the oven to 250°F and line a baking sheet with parchment.
2. Place the almonds in a large bowl.
3. Add the olive oil, cinnamon, and salt then toss to coat.
4. Spread the almonds on the baking sheet and roast for 1 hour.

5. Remove from the oven and cool slightly to serve warm or cool completely and store in an airtight container.

Lemon Blueberry Cupcakes

Nutrition Facts (Per Serving): Calories: 210, Carbs: 20g, Fat: 13g, Protein: 1g

Servings: 12

Ingredients:

- ½ cup sifted coconut flour
- ¼ teaspoon baking soda
- ¼ teaspoon salt
- 6 large eggs, whisked
- ½ cup coconut oil
- ¼ cup honey
- 2 tablespoons lemon juice
- 1 tablespoon fresh lemon zest
- ½ cup fresh blueberries

Instructions:

1. Preheat the oven to 350°F and line a regular muffin pan with paper liners.
2. Combine the coconut flour, baking soda, and salt in a food processor.
3. Pulse several times then add the eggs, coconut oil, honey, lemon juice, and lemon zest.
4. Blend smooth then stir in the blueberries and divide the batter evenly in the pan.
5. Bake for 20 to 24 minutes until a knife inserted in the center comes out clean.
6. Cool the cupcakes for 1 hour then frost as desired.

Grilled Balsamic Peaches

Nutrition Facts (Per Serving): Calories: 172, Carbs: 26g, Fat: 6g, Protein: 5g

Servings: 4

Ingredients:

- 4 ripe peaches
- Balsamic vinegar, as needed

Instructions:

1. Slice the peaches in half and remove the pits.
2. Preheat a grill pan to medium-low heat and spray with cooking spray.
3. Place the peaches cut-side-down on the grill and cook for 3 to 5 minutes until they just start to soften.
4. Transfer the grilled peaches to serving bowls and drizzle with balsamic vinegar to serve.

Maple Walnut Trail Mix

Nutrition Facts (Per Serving): Calories: 278, Carbs: 28g, Fat: 15g, Protein: 7g

Servings: 8 to 10

Ingredients:

- 2 cups walnut halves
- 2 cups whole almonds
- 1 cup whole cashews
- 1 cup hulled sunflower seeds
- 1 cup seedless raisings
- ¼ cup pure maple syrup
- ¼ cup melted coconut oil
- 1 teaspoon almond extract

- 1 teaspoon ground cinnamon

Instructions:

1. Preheat the oven to 350°F and line a rimmed baking sheet with parchment.
2. Combine the nuts, seeds, and raisins in a large bowl.
3. In a separate bowl, whisk together the remaining ingredients.
4. Drizzle the wet mixture over the nuts and seeds then toss to coat.
5. Spread the mixture evenly on the prepared baking sheet.
6. Bake for 15 to 20 minutes until browned.
7. Let the trail mix cool completely then store in an airtight container.

Coconut Almond Chia Pudding

Nutrition Facts (Per Serving): Calories: 201, Carbs: 23g, Fat: 10g, Protein: 6g

Servings: 3

Ingredients:

- 1 ½ cups unsweetened coconut milk
- 8 pitted Medjool dates
- ¼ cup unsweetened cocoa powder
- ¼ cup chia seeds
- 1 teaspoon almond extract

Instructions:

1. Combine the coconut milk, dates, cocoa powder, chia seeds, and almond extract in a blender.
2. Blend on high speed for 30 to 60 seconds, scraping down the sides as needed, until smooth and well combined.
3. Spoon into dessert cups and chill until ready to serve.

Baked Beet Chips

Nutrition Facts (Per Serving): Calories: 60, Carbs: 8g, Fat: 3g, Protein: 1g

Servings: 4

Ingredients:

- 5 whole beets, peeled
- Olive oil, as needed
- Salt and pepper

Instructions:

1. Preheat the oven to 175°F and line two baking sheets with parchment.
2. Slice the beets as thinly as possible and arrange them on the baking sheet in a single layer.
3. Drizzle with oil and season with salt and pepper then bake for 20 to 25 minutes, turning the tray halfway through.
4. Turn off the oven and let the slices cool until crisp then store in an airtight container.

Conclusion

If you've been diagnosed with diabetes, it is up to you to take your health into your own hands. Making healthy changes to your diet and lifestyle can greatly improve your condition and, in the case of type 2 diabetes, may reverse it entirely. Keep in mind, however, that it takes time to make lasting changes so commit yourself to following the paleo diet and do your best to stick to it. The information provided in this book should help you to gain a comprehensive understanding of the diet as well as tips for getting started.

Diabetes is a serious condition that can lead to some pretty devastating consequences if left untreated. If you have diabetes, do yourself a favor and start getting it under control sooner than later. When you're ready to step up and make a change, follow the tips in this book and give some of the tasty paleo recipes a try!

Finally, thank you very much for taking the time to read this book. We sincerely hope you have gained something of value. We are here to serve you and every encouragement from you means a lot to us.

If you enjoyed this book, please be kind enough to leave a review and let us know what you liked about it. Your support really does make a difference and I read all the reviews personally so can I understand what my readers particularly enjoyed and then feature more of that in future books.

Index

Almond Butter Brownies	72
Apple Walnut Chicken Salad	43
Avocado Deviled Eggs	70
Avocado Egg Salad	41
Avocado Spinach Salad with Egg	42
Bacon-Wrapped Turkey Breast	63
Baked Beet Chips	77
Baked Cinnamon Apple Chips	70
Balsamic Grilled Salmon	54
Blueberry Coconut Smoothie	25
Cajun Chicken and Veggies	62
Chicken Tikka Masala	60
Chocolate Almond Butter Smoothie	37
Chocolate Chia Pudding	71
Chopped Chicken and Mango Salad	45
Cilantro Lime Chicken	67
Cinnamon Coconut Flour Waffles	35
Cinnamon Roasted Nuts	73
Coco-Vanilla Chia Pudding	31
Coconut Almond Chia Pudding	76
Cream of Broccoli Soup	44
Creamy Avocado Walnut Smoothie	34
Creamy Cucumber Dill Salad	47
Curried Butternut Squash Soup	40
Curry Grilled Pork Chops	68
Easy Chicken and Vegetable Soup	49
Easy Garlic Shrimp	63
Grilled Balsamic Peaches	75
Grilled Salmon with Mango Sauce	64
Ham and Red Pepper Frittata	27
Hearty Beef and Vegetable Stew	44
Herb-Crusted Lamb Chops	58
Herb-Roasted Pork Tenderloin	54
Lamb and Root Vegetable Stew	48
Lemon Blueberry Cupcakes	74
Lemon Chicken with Broccoli	65
Light & Fluffy Banana Protein Pancake	33
Maple Country Style Pork Ribs	66
Maple Walnut Trail Mix	75
Meatloaf with BBQ Sauce	57
Mixed Vegetable Frittata	36
Mushroom and Leek Soup	46
Pumpkin Protein Pancakes	28
Raspberry Kale Smoothie	32
Roasted Tomato Basil Soup	41
Rosemary Roasted Chicken	52
Seared Scallops with Herb Butter	56
Sesame Kale Chips	72
Slow Cooker Balsamic Roast Beef	61
Slow Cooker Pulled Pork	55
Spiced Apple Walnut Muffins	26
Spiced Pumpkin Soup	50
Spinach and Mushroom Omelet	31
Strawberry Ginger Beet Smoothie	29
Sweet Potato Breakfast Skillet	30
Thai Coconut Vegetable Curry	53
Tomato Basil Omelet	25
Triple Berry Smoothie	36
Vegetable Egg White Omelet	34
Zucchini Pasta and Meatballs	59

How To Get The Color Paperback Version

1. Go to Amazon.com
2. Search for the book title: Paleo Diet Cookbook For Diabetics With Color Pictures (by Barbara Trisler)
3. The relevant book will appear in the search result.
4. Click on the option you prefer (kindle or paperback) and make your purchase.

How To Get The Bonus Recipe Image Booklet

1. Go to www.MillenniumPublishingLimited.com
2. Navigate to the tab labeled "Barbara Trisler" (hover over it)
3. Click on "Paleo Diet Cookbook Recipe Image Booklet"
4. Specify where you want to receive the recipe image booklet

Made in the USA
Middletown, DE
03 December 2019